Dialysis Advice
A Patient's Point Of View

Kathleen Russell

Copyright 2013
Walrus Productions
4805 N.E. 106th Street
Seattle, WA 98125
206-364-4365

Photos by Larry Wall
Layout Design: The Durland Group

This book was printed in the USA

ISBN - 978-1470120283

10 9 8 7 6 5 4 3

I dedicate this book to all the current and future dialysis patients. I want to acknowledge all the generous donors who have given financial support to the Northwest Kidney Centers. You are the unsung heroes.

My deepest appreciation goes to the nurses, technicians, and staff members for having chosen a career that saves and extends the lives of their patients.

A special thanks to: Catherine Burr, Margie Norman, and Munya Souaiaia for their priceless assistance.

I especially want to acknowledge the extraordinary hours of editing contribution by my dear friend, Christine Adkins. Your dedication and invaluable expertise is appreciated beyond words. You helped "unscramble the eggs" with a flair, love, and professionalism. I am so grateful to have you in my life.

I can't send this book off to print without also acknowledging my hubby, Larry Wall. You are the powerhouse behind this production and although you may prefer to "hide in the weeds" when it comes to authoring this book, we both know this was your idea. Your relentless writing, interviewing, and rearranging of pages is what made this book possible. Your enthusiasm for envisioning this book and the heart that you put into it have made me love you even more.

Kathleen Russell

Table of Contents

INTRODUCTION

Many years ago, being dependent on hemodialysis was a thought that would never have crossed my mind. Today, it is a crucial part of my daily routine, both life saving and life changing. In 2009, I made a YouTube video of a nine-minute condensed version of one of my dialysis procedures. My objective was to help people facing the possibility of traveling this same road, and the response from patients, family, techs, and nurses was so positive, I was motivated to take it a step farther. This book is the result. It is my personal perspective of this lifesaving process, and I hope that it will give new patients a glimpse of what they should expect as well as how to take an active role in their care.

The advice I am offering in this book is a reflection of my personal experience and is intended to assist those who are currently having hemodialysis treatments or about to start. Dialysis is not easy, but this information may give you a much clearer understanding of the process and may also change the way you feel about it. Staying positive and finding new ways to combat the negatives just might make it a whole lot easier.

Please Note:
This book focuses on hemodialysis because it is the treatment my nephrologist and I agreed would be right for me. There are other treatment regimens that you may wish to discuss with your own doctor in order to make the best decision for your individual situation. A general explanation of the primary options is provided on page 26, but anything more than a brief description is beyond the scope of this book. Talk with your physician about the choices that are available to you.

WATCH MY EDUCATIONAL VIDEO

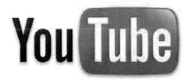

Enter "Dialysis Treatment Procedure" in the YouTube search bar to watch the video below.

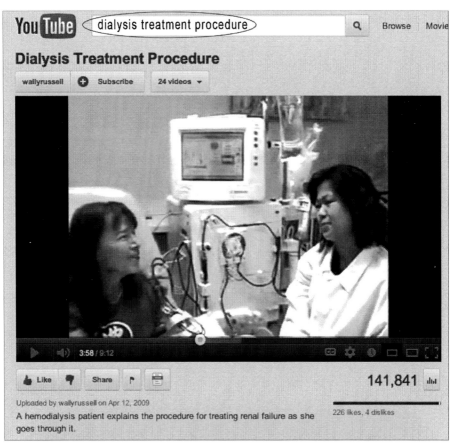

Watch Kathleen demonstrate and explain her dialysis.

KIDNEY FUNCTIONS

To understand what happens when your kidneys fail, it is important to understand all that they normally do for you:

- Make urine.

- Remove wastes and extra fluid from your blood.

- Control your body's electrolyte balance (potassium, sodium, chloride, and bicarbonate).

- Help control your blood pressure.

- Keep bones healthy by balancing phosphorus and calcium.

- Make more red blood cells by producing EPO (erythropoietin), a hormone that stimulates your bone marrow to produce more red blood cells.

KIDNEY FAILURE

The following conditions result when the kidneys stop functioning properly:

- Waste products build up in the blood, a condition known as uremia. Having regular dialysis treatments and limiting foods that contain sodium, potassium, and phosphorus can mitigate most of the problems associated with uremia.

- Anemia is common because the damaged kidneys slow the production of the hormone EPO, which helps the bone marrow make red blood cells.

- Amyloidosis results when abnormal protein in the blood (amyloid) is deposited in tissues and organs, including joints and tendons. This can cause pain, stiffness, and fluid in the joints.

- Far higher rates of heart and blood vessel problems occur.

- Insomnia, restless legs, and cramping may occur.

- Itchy skin is a common complaint of those receiving hemodialysis.

- Psychological and emotional reactions to kidney failure occur as well as physical ones. Depression can be an issue, but it can often be treated with adjustments to the diet or dialysis schedule, counseling, or medication. Discuss your concerns with your health care provider.

Sometimes side effects from required medications can trigger adverse reactions due to the drugs themselves or as a result of interactions with other medications. Dizziness and constipation, for example, are common. Hopefully, these negative side effects are outweighed by the benefits of taking a particular drug. Again, always discuss your concerns with your doctor.

WHAT WENT WRONG?

My path to kidney failure was different than most. I had a rare condition called microscopic polyarteritis nodosa, which caused my body's immune system to begin to attack my own kidneys. For two years, I experienced chronic pain and dealt with it by taking Ibuprofen frequently. At that time, I was unaware that most painkillers such as Ibuprofen and aspirin can be hard on the kidneys. When I was finally given a urine test, my protein and blood counts were off the charts, leading to five years of chemotherapy. Unfortunately, chemotherapy along with the dyes hospitals use for certain tests, colonoscopy prep liquids, enemas, certain medications, and many minerals found in vitamins can stress the kidneys, and they all took a serious toll. As my kidneys began to fail, I lost my appetite, and when I did eat, I would often throw up. I lost muscle mass as well as weight, and I suffered from exhaustion from which there was no relief. I finally recognized how serious things were when the only way I could manage the short flight of stairs to my bedroom was to crawl on my hands and knees. I don't know whether or not I was clinically depressed, but there was little I could do beyond lying in bed, and I had lost interest in what was going on around me. It was at that point that I reluctantly started occasional hospital visits for dialysis. I began weekly EPO shots (erythropoietin – a hormone produced by the kidneys that stimulates the bone marrow to produce more red blood cells). Every week, I would read my lab reports and I soon became aware that eating less protein, potassium, phosphorus, and sodium slowed down the deterioration of my kidneys as well. This was something I could do for myself. I watched my creatinine number level off or sometimes even drop because of careful dietary monitoring, and because I was so vigilant about what I ate, I was able to give myself a few years before initiating treatments.

BEGINNING DIALYSIS

From the time I first started experiencing kidney problems to the point where I required regular dialysis it had been 11 years. It finally became clear, however, that the inevitable had been delayed as long as it could, and I was scheduled for my first dialysis treatment at the kidney center.

My first treatment did not go well. It was very unfortunate that I was so unprepared for the violent leg cramps I experienced. Sobbing, I vowed to the nurse that I was never coming back, knowing full well what that would mean. In the days that followed, I shared several tearful conversations with my closest friends about my decision to die.

Despite the difficulties of that first experience, a few more months of decline brought me back to the kidney center for another round of dialysis. Thankfully, it went much better, and I began receiving treatments every 10-12 days. I also started to learn more about what had caused my severe leg cramps, how to "uncramp" by doing opposite stretches, and how to avoid them almost altogether by determining a more accurate "dry weight." For me, taking off more than 1.5 kg fluid at that time was more likely to cause cramping.

As time has gone by, I have had to increase dialysis, first to once a week, and then to twice a week because my CO_2 was so low, and my body was becoming too acidic. I continue to monitor my dry weight gain, and currently my upper limit of fluid removal is at 1.7 kg. I have learned how important it is to get to know my body and listen to what it tells me.

Although my situation was rare, kidney failure can result from a variety of more common conditions including high blood pressure, e. coli, a genetic disease called polycystic kidney disease, or sometimes an injury. In approximately 45 percent of cases, however, kidney failure is the result of diabetes. This is such an insidious disease, and too many people ignore the warning signs. If you are a borderline diabetic or have diabetes, I can't overemphasize how important it is to take action now and work closely with a good doctor to manage your blood glucose levels. With a structured regular diet and exercise, you may be able to delay dialysis or possibly avoid it.

The more you understand what's happening to your body, the better, and educating yourself about your kidneys is sure to be an ongoing process. Knowing how to strictly monitor your health, and your diet in particular, is central to the treatment of your kidney failure. Having a life-threatening illness can make you feel powerless, but information is power:

- Keep a notebook where you can write down your questions before appointments with your doctor.

- Be sure to ask for clarification if there is something you do not understand.

- Record the answers while you are with your doctor.

I can't tell you how many times I have come home after an appointment without having written the answers to my questions in my notebook, because I was so certain I would remember it all. I've learned the hard way to always write everything down. I would strongly encourage you to do the same, so you can keep the information as a permanent reference.

In addition to keeping your notebook, start learning the basic lab terminology and what it means. Not only will this help you in your conversations with your doctor, but it will also help you to use your monthly lab reports to monitor your diet.

During my pre-dialysis years in particular, I maintained a line graph of my hematocrit, creatinine, and BUN (blood, urea, nitrogen). After starting dialysis, I became focused on my eKt/V, dry weight, potassium, hemoglobin, hematocrit, phosphorus, and PTH levels. The graph and lab reports continue to serve as my guide to the adjustments that I periodically need to make to my diet. Look carefully at your own monthly results and make sure you understand them.

My doctor recommended I get a digital scale so I could monitor and manage my weight gain between dialysis sessions. Most patients have limited or no ability to urinate, so if you notice a significant gain, cut back drastically on sodium intake and reduce fluids. The less you gain, the less trauma your body will feel during dialysis because you won't have to have as much fluid removed to achieve your "dry weight."

If you take advantage of every opportunity to learn as much as you possibly can, you will have far more options for being in a position of control. Learn to look after yourself. No one can do this as well as you can, and the sooner you start, the better your chances will be to delay the necessity for dialysis.

THE IMPORTANCE OF DIET
What is the relationship between hemodialysis and diet?

Food gives you energy and helps your body repair itself. After it is broken down in your stomach and intestines, the blood picks up nutrients from the digested food and carries them to all your body cells. The cells absorb these nutrients and put waste products back into the bloodstream. When your kidneys are healthy, they work around the clock to filter wastes from your blood, which then leave your body when you urinate. Other wastes are removed in bowel movements.

When your kidneys stop working, hemodialysis will remove wastes from your blood. But between dialysis sessions, wastes can build up in your blood and make you sick. You can reduce the amount of wastes by watching what you eat and drink, so a good meal plan is very important if you want to improve your dialysis and your health.

What do I need to know about calories?

Calories provide energy for your body. If your doctor recommends it, you may need to reduce your calories, but other people on dialysis may need to gain weight. This may mean finding ways to add calories to your diet. Vegetable oils like olive oil, canola oil, and safflower oil are good sources of calories. Use them generously on breads, rice, and noodles. This is the healthiest way to add fat to your diet if you need to gain weight. Butter and margarines are rich in calories, but these fatty foods can also clog your arteries. Use them less often. Hard candy, sugar, honey, jam, and jelly provide calories and energy without clogging arteries or adding other things that your body does not need.

What do I need to know about protein?

A healthy diet is important to dialysis patients because it strengthens your resistance to infections as well as improves your recovery time should you need surgery. Protein in particular helps you to keep muscle as well as repair tissue, but not all proteins are equal. When protein breaks down in your body, it produces waste products called urea. If urea builds up in your blood, it is a sign that your kidneys are struggling. For this reason, eating as much high-quality protein as possible is important: higher quality equals less waste and happier kidneys! Good sources of high-quality protein include meat, fish, poultry, and eggs (especially egg whites). I take an amino acid tablet daily to help keep my albumin level above the desired minimum of 4.0. Choose organic foods, if that is an option available to you.

What do I need to know about fluids?

You really need to watch how much you drink. Fluid can build up between dialysis sessions, causing swelling and weight gain. Overloading your system with fluid affects your blood pressure, makes your heart work harder, and could lead to serious heart trouble. Controlling your thirst and thereby controlling your fluid intake is a simple but very important way to be directly involved in your own care. It is important to be aware that you "eat" water as well as drink it. Foods that are liquid at room temperature (soup, Jell-O, and ice cream) contain water, and many fruits and vegetables contain large amounts of water too. Melons, grapes, apples, oranges, tomatoes, lettuce, and celery are especially high and will add to your fluid intake.

You can keep your fluids down by drinking from smaller cups or glasses. Some people like to chew on ice chips. Both give the satisfaction of drinking without creating thirst.

Your "dry weight" is how much you weigh after a dialysis session when all of the extra fluid in your body has been removed. If you let too much fluid build up between sessions, it is harder to get down to your proper dry weight. Talk with your doctor regularly about what your dry weight should be. Ultimately, you should become the best judge for establishing your dry weight because you know what you are eating and drinking, and whether you are having cramps at night or during dialysis.

What do I need to know about sodium?

The best way to reduce fluid intake is to reduce thirst caused by the salt you eat. Sodium is found in salt and most of the foods we eat. Be careful to choose low-sodium products and avoid processed and packaged products like canned foods and frozen dinners which can contain large amounts of sodium. Too much sodium makes you thirsty. If you drink too much fluid, your heart has to work harder to pump that fluid through your body. Over time, this can cause high blood pressure and congestive heart failure. Try to eat fresh foods that are naturally low in sodium and look for products labeled low-sodium. Do not use salt substitutes because they contain potassium. Talk with your facility's dietitian about flavoring your food with spices and managing your thirst. Remember, following a low-salt diet can delay kidney failure.

What do I need to know about phosphorus?

Phosphorus is a mineral found in many foods including dairy products, dried beans, peas, colas, and nuts. Too much phosphorus in your blood pulls calcium from your bones, which will make them more likely to break. Too much phosphorus may also make your skin itch. Foods like milk and cheese are high in this mineral, so people on dialysis are usually limited to a 1/2 cup of milk per day. The renal dietitian can give you more specific information regarding management of phosphorus levels in the foods you eat. In addition, you will probably need to take a phosphate binder like Renagel, PhosLo, Renvela, Tums, or calcium carbonate to control the phosphorus in your blood between dialysis sessions. These medications bind with phosphorus and are then removed by passing through the stool.

What do I need to know about potassium?

Potassium is a mineral found in many foods especially milk, fruit, and vegetables. It affects how steadily your heart beats. Healthy kidneys keep the right amount of potassium in the blood to keep the heart beating at a steady pace, but if your potassium levels rise between dialysis sessions, it can affect your heartbeat. Consuming too much potassium can be *very dangerous* to your heart and may even cause death.

To control potassium levels in your blood, avoid foods like avocados, bananas, kiwis, and dried fruit, which are very high in this mineral. Eat smaller portions of other high-potassium foods. For example, eat half a pear instead of a whole pear. Eat only very small portions of oranges and melons. Let your lab results be your guide.

As you can see, what you put into your body is critical to your kidney function. Everyone is unique and their reasons for needing dialysis may differ, so be sure to follow the prescribed dialysis treatment orders given by your doctor and meet with your facility dietitian regarding your dialysis diet.

As part of your diet, you must limit your fluid intake. Always keep in mind that fluids are not just in what you drink but in varying amounts in everything you eat. Although I don't consider my diet a super strict one, I carefully monitor what I eat and you should too. Here's what works for me:

I now start off each day with *Juice Plus*® capsules. Although you should always get your doctor's approval before taking supplements, I have found that they really help me maintain a proper potassium balance that allows me to eat more fruits and vegetables.

My diet has gone through changes as my disease has progressed. I have learned to focus on those things I can eat and enjoy rather than dwelling on what I can't. The key is a **small portion** and this is a rule you should follow with everything you eat. If I get hungry between meals, little snacks of toast, nuts, or celery with peanut butter help me to fill the gap. I never miss a little pick-me-up with my afternoon tea. For dinner, I'll treat myself to a wide variety of meals, but in very small portions. I eat a lot of white rice and limit potatoes to once a month. Fruit and vegetables get cut back when my potassium gets too high but on the days before dialysis, I will sometimes give myself permission to splurge and eat a little more of the "bad stuff." I don't do this very often but when I do, I figure that's the best time.

When in doubt, remember to follow the small portions rule with everything you eat.

VASCULAR ACCESS FOR HEMODIALYSIS

One important step before starting regular hemodialysis sessions is preparing a vascular access, the site on your body where blood is removed and returned during treatments.

The three basic kinds of vascular access for hemodialysis are an arteriovenous or AV fistula, an AV graft, and a venous catheter. An AV fistula is useful because it causes the vein to grow larger and stronger for easy access to the blood system. It is considered the best long-term vascular access for hemodialysis because it provides adequate blood flow, lasts a long time, and has a lower complication rate than other types of access. If an AV fistula cannot be created, an AV graft or venous catheter may be needed.

Vascular access requires surgery a couple of months before you start using it for dialysis. Once your fistula surgery is complete, you should be able to put your finger on it and feel what is called a *thrill*. This thrill is a kind of buzzing sensation felt by pressing a finger on your fistula. What you are feeling is the turbulence of the blood, and that lets you know that your fistula is working. It could be compared to two rivers running into each other from different directions.

You should check to be sure you can feel the thrill several times a day. If at any time you can't feel it, you should go immediately to the emergency room for a heparin flush in order to preserve your fistula.

Protect your fistula. Bags with handles should be carried by hand - not over your fistula arm. Do not allow anyone to take your blood pressure on your fistula arm, avoid sleeping on it, and make sure the people around you are aware of the need for you to protect it.

What is an arteriovenous fistula?

An AV fistula requires advanced planning because after surgery, a fistula takes a while to develop; (mine took two months). The advantage is that a properly formed fistula is less likely to form clots or become infected than other kinds of vascular access. Properly formed fistulas also tend to last many years longer than any other kind of vascular access.

A surgeon can create an AV fistula by connecting an artery directly to a vein, frequently in the forearm. This causes more blood to flow into the vein, which then grows larger and stronger, making repeated needle insertions for hemodialysis treatments easier.

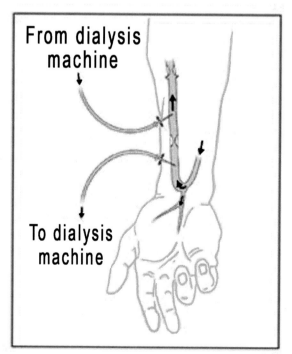

Forearm arteriovenous fistula

What is an arteriovenous graft?

If you have small veins that won't develop properly into a fistula, you can get a vascular access that connects an artery to a vein using a synthetic tube, or graft, implanted under the skin in your arm. The graft becomes an artificial vein that can be used repeatedly for needle placement and blood access during hemodialysis. A graft doesn't need to develop as a fistula does, so it can be used sooner after placement, often within two or three weeks. Compared with properly formed fistulas, grafts tend to have more problems with clotting and infection and need replacement sooner. However, a well cared for graft can last several years. Having a graft does not eliminate the discomfort of having needles inserted.

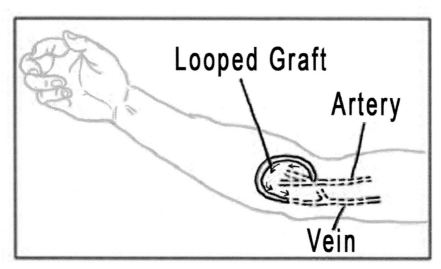

One kind of AV graft

What is a venous catheter for temporary access?

If your kidney disease has progressed quickly, you may not have time to get a permanent vascular access before you start hemodialysis treatments. You may need to use a venous catheter as a temporary access.

A catheter is a tube inserted into a vein in your neck, chest, or leg near the groin. It has two chambers to allow a two-way flow of blood. Once a catheter is placed, needle insertion is not necessary. You will have two exterior short tubes stitched and taped in place, which connect to the heart. Hookup to the dialysis machine is quick and painless. Having such a catheter can be somewhat restrictive and sometimes uncomfortable. When I had one, I had a hard time learning to sleep on my back instead of on my side or stomach.

Catheters are not ideal for permanent access. They can clog, become infected, and cause narrowing of the veins in which they are placed. If you need to start hemodialysis immediately, a catheter will work for several weeks or months while your permanent access develops.

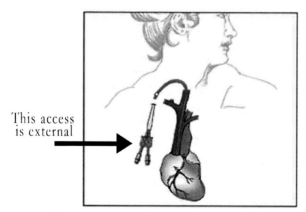

This access is external

Venous catheter for temporary hemodialysis access

Use EMLA cream to numb needle insertion sites.

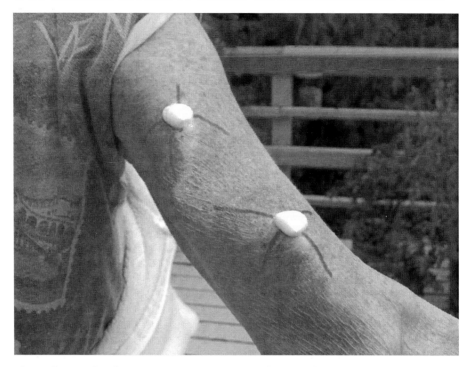

One hour before my start time, I have found it helps me to apply two dots of EMLA cream to the needle insertion sites on my fistula. Using a washable felt pen, I then mark the spot with an X, so I can rotate the insertion points slightly up and down with each treatment. This allows the technician to hit the right spot and gives my arm time to heal. Some patients use the "buttonhole" method (always using the same insertion point), but it usually requires having the same technician each time you have a treatment.

Some people elect to have lidocaine shots instead of using the EMLA cream, but I prefer the cream because there is less scarring. Of course there are those who don't use anything at all, and my hat goes off to them. I'm not quite that macho.

If you get injections of EPO or lidocaine, ask the nurse to give you the injection SLOWLY, as (for me) it reduces the sting.

ABOUT THE MACHINE

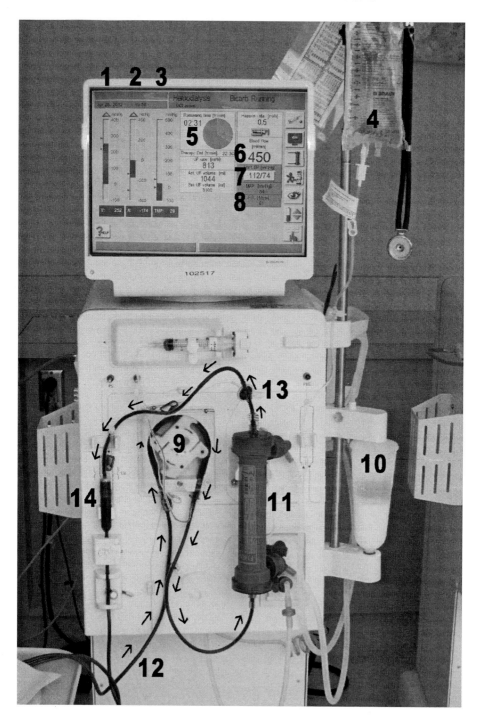

1. **Venous Pressure**

2. **Arterial Pressure**

3. **Transmembrane Pressure**

4. **Saline Solution**

5. **Time Remaining**

6. **Pump Speed**

7. **Blood Pressure**

8. **Pulse Rate**

9. **Pump**

10. **Bicarbonate**

11. **Dialyzer Filter**

12. **Blood From You**

13. **Blood Back To You**

14. **Venous Drip Bulb**

ALTERNATIVE TREATMENTS

Kidney Transplant: It may take years to make it to the top of the transplant waiting list, unless you are fortunate enough to have a living donor willing to donate a kidney. Poor matches are much more likely to be rejected by your body, so there are numerous tests both the donor and recipient must go through to determine the best match possible.

Peritoneal Dialysis: In this process, tubing is surgically implanted in the abdomen, and the peritoneal cavity is bathed with diasylate to flush away wastes. It allows for home treatment, but it will necessitate having adequate space to store the boxes of diasylate that will be shipped to you on a regular basis. There are two types of peritoneal dialysis: Continuous Ambulatory Peritoneal Dialysis (CAPD) or Continuous Cycler-assisted Peritoneal Dialysis (CCPD). CAPD can be done manually, but CCPD requires a machine called a cycler to fill and drain your abdomen, which can be done while you sleep.

Home Hemodialysis: If home hemodialysis is your choice, you most likely will start out at a facility and then go through a training program until you are proficient enough to be on your own. This is an advantage for more active people who have help available to them in case of an emergency or to assist with inserting the needles. I know of patients who love to travel in their RVs, and they have portable dialysis machines that they take with them in order to stay consistent with their treatments.

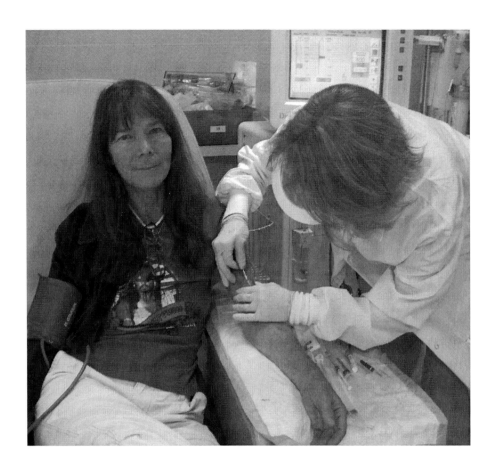

Dialysis… it's not the most fun thing to have to do, but make the best of it. Dialysis is a *Life Support System.*
So keep your chin up.

- Kathleen Russell

PROBLEMS I'VE HAD

FISTULAS – My first fistula was surgically created near my left wrist. The first time it was used, a dialysis tech had difficulty getting the needles into my tiny, rolling veins. When he finished, he said he was going to try to make it a little bigger, put a blood pressure cuff on my arm just above the fistula, and pumped the cuff up. My fistula immediately ballooned out and I heard him mutter to my husband, "I think I ruined her fistula." No "thrill" could be detected and I was rushed down to surgery. (Fortunately this happened in the hospital.) They tried to flush out the fistula with heparin but it was too late. The doctors put me back on a chest catheter.

When I finally started regular dialysis with my new fistula, the techs still had difficulty with the needle insertions in my tiny, rolling veins, and I had frequent "infiltrations" where the needle would go all the way through the vein. This was painful and caused immediate swelling and ugly bruising. Finally, my surgeon suggested putting a fistula in my upper arm where my veins were larger. After the initial healing from that surgery, I started lifting hand weights and my fistula grew strong and plump - not attractive, but it is much easier for the techs to insert the needles and access with accuracy.

ITCHING – Itching is a common complaint among dialysis patients although not all patients are troubled by it. While it's hard to know the exact cause(s), itching may be brought about by dry skin, high phosphorus levels, allergic reactions, high blood levels of parathyroid hormone (PTH), or sensitivity to the tape used to secure your needles.

I get "the itchies" during and especially at the end of my dialysis run. I think I am allergic to something in the diasylate, and my skin is very sensitive to the adhesive tape used to secure the needles in my arm. My solution is to carry cotton balls and a bottle of *Sea Breeze*® astringent along with me to apply to my arm as necessary for relief. In addition, my doctor prescribed hydroxyzine pills to take before I go in for treatment. They seem to help as well.

CRAMPING – From my experience, there are two causes for cramping during hemodialysis: removing too much fluid and removing the fluid too fast. When too much fluid is removed, it results in dehydration, and muscle cramping of the hands, feet, and legs is fairly common. At times severe, this can occur near the end of dialysis and persist for a time even after the procedure is completed. If your blood pressure is low, you may be given normal saline to increase the fluid in your body, which will often relieve symptoms. You may also be given hypertonic saline or glucose, and a medication such as quinine is sometimes prescribed for chronic leg cramps. Heat and massage can help provide relief as well.

Your two best defenses against muscle cramping are maintaining a balance between your dry weight and fluid gains and avoiding foods that make you thirsty and elevate your fluid intake. Be sure to stick to your daily fluid and sodium restrictions. Going to dialysis with less fluid means they won't need to take off too much too quickly. Cramping can be a guide to establishing your dry weight. If you have persistent cramping, you might try "upping your dry weight." Try to stretch out of a cramp, or if you can carefully stand up, that often helps. (If I get cramps in the middle of the night, I've found that the best way to get relief is to get out of bed quickly and walk around.)

BLEEDING AND BRUISING – My skin has become very thin and just the slightest scratching will cause bleeding under the skin, leaving marks on my arm. I bleed easily from routine cuts and scratches and it takes a while to get the bleeding to stop. I surmise that this is because I am given heparin (an anti-clotting agent) every time I do dialysis.

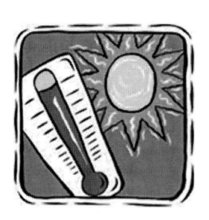 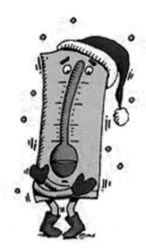

TOO HOT / TOO COLD? – Most patients don't know this, but if your blood pressure isn't too low, you may be allowed to have your technician change your blood temperature up or down one degree with a quick adjustment of the dialysis machine. It can make a huge difference in your comfort.

I always get cold during my dialysis treatments, resulting from the overhead air circulation ducts that blow towards my chair. I sometimes use a privacy screen to block the cold draft. Some dialysis centers have heated chairs and overhead heat. Blankets, leg warmers, or long underwear can help keep you warm too.

If you tend to get too hot, it helps to wear loose fitting clothes or removable layers.

LAB RESULTS

Knowing exactly what your labs mean and taking action is a must for maintaining a healthy living condition.

LAB TEST	YOUR NUMBER	YOUR GOAL	COMMENTS
Potassium (K+)	5.3	3.5 - 5.5	> Mineral found in fruits, vegetables, other foods. > Affects how your muscles work, including your heart > Too high or too low can affect your heart beats > Treated with dialysis, diet, and medication
Albumin	4.6	4 or higher	> Made in your body from protein > If too low, your body can't heal or fight infection well > Treated with diet, supplements, and dialysis
Hemoglobin (Hgb)	11.2	10 - 12	> The part of red blood cells that carries oxygen throughout your body > If too low, you are anemic and can feel very tired and have other symptoms. > Treated with Epogen or Aranesp and iron
Iron %Saturation	69	More than 20%	> How much iron is available in your body > Needed to make red blood cells > Treated with IV iron medication
Calcium (Ca++)	10.0	8.5 - 10.2	> Mineral that healthy kidneys balance with phosphorus > If out of balance, can affect heart, blood vessel, and bone health > Treated with diet and medications (binders)
Phosphorus (PO4-)	(5.9)	3.5 - 5.5	> Mineral that healthy kidneys balance with calcium > If out of balance, can affect heart, blood vessel, and bone health > Treated with dialysis, diet and medications (binders)
PTH (parathyroid hormone)	143	150 - 300	> The messenger that controls the movement of calcium and phosphorus in your body > Affect heart, blood vessel and bone health > Controlled with diet and vitamin D medication
spKT/V (dialysis adequacy: if you dialyze 3 or less times a week)	1.8847	1.4 or higher	> Measures how well waste is being removed by dialysis > If too low, affects your long term health and survival
Dry Weight	58.0 05/07/2012		> Your body's weight without extra fluid > Should be your weight at the end of dialysis treatment > If you are not reaching your dry weight, you are at higher risk for strokes, heart attacks, and heart failure
HgbA1C		Less than 7%	> For diabetics > Measures how well you controlled your blood sugar over last 2-3 months

The hemodialysis lab results (above) show that "Phosphorus" is high. In this case, the patient most likely needs more binders and fewer dairy products.

KEEP A CURRENT LIST OF YOUR MEDS

Staying on top of your labs and meds will help you immensely.

I highly recommend always keeping an up-to-date list of your medications handy. Like me, you will have to take a vast number of different pills, and it is a challenge to remember them all. It will be much easier for you, as well as for those who are providing your care, if you always have a current list of medications available. In addition, make sure your loved ones and anyone responsible for your care knows where this list is kept in case of an emergency.

Some examples:

- Copy for dialysis unit each time there's a change in meds.

- Copy for every doctor's visit.

- Copy for dentist.

- Copy to take to hospital.

- Copy for home.

- Copy when taking trips.

MY DAILY MEDICATIONS

NAME	FREQ	DOSAGE
AMBIEN	1 per Day	10mg (sleep aid)
AMINO ACIDS	1 per Day	1000mg (augment protein)
CLONAZEPAM	2 1/2 per Day	5mg (anti-anxiety)
DOCUSATE SODIUM	2 per Day	250mg (stool softener)
VITAMIN D3	1 per Day	5000 IU per
FOSRENOL	1 per Day	1000mg (phosphorus binder)
HYDROXYZINE	50mg (for itching from dialysis)	
KIONEX	1/4 C in water (If high potassium symptoms occur)	
LEVOTHYROXINE	1 per Day	1.37mcg (for thyroid condition)
LIDOCAINE/PRILOCN	30g (EMLA)	(numbing cream for needles)
LOSARTAN POTASSIUM	2 per Day	50 mg (blood pressure)
METOPROLOL TARTRATE	2 per day	25 mg (blood pressure)
NEPHROVITE	1 per Day (special vitamin for kidney failure)	
OMEGA 3	2 per Day	(good for heart)
RENVELA	8 per Day	800mg (phosphorus binder)
SENSIPAR	2 per Day	60mg (to decrease PTH)
TUMS	6 per Day	(phosphorus binder)
EPO, ZEMPLAR, IRON	Injections with Dialysis	

JUICE PLUS CAPSULES   6 per Day (fruit and vegetable capsules to help maintain potassium balance and improve nutrition)

TRAVEL TIPS

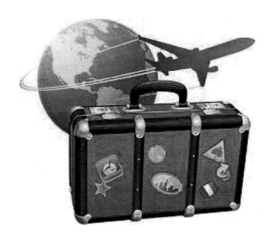

There are over 5,000 dialysis facilities around the country but if you are traveling, it is important to start planning and making arrangements at least six to eight weeks in advance. More time should be allowed when traveling to popular vacation spots during holidays. Your dialysis facility should have an experienced staff member who can help you arrange for dialysis treatments away from home.

Be aware that some dialysis facilities have different rules and it might be wise to ask about them before making your plans. Some may not allow a spouse or visitor to accompany you during treatment, while others may not allow you to eat.

If you are traveling overseas, keep all your pills in the original prescription bottles. It is also essential to have a letter from your doctor that states that the drugs you have in your possession are "life sustaining," or the customs officers could take them from you. Again, whether you are traveling overseas or just a few miles away, always have your list of all your medications, just in case of an emergency or any unforeseen circumstances.

TRANSPORTATION ISSUES

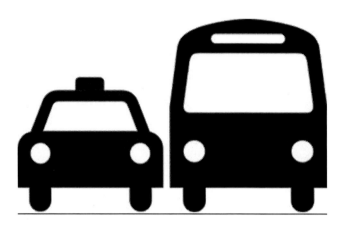

TRANSPORTATION

Patients travel to dialysis in a number of ways including taxis, wheelchair vans, passenger vans, and buses, but approximately one-quarter come to dialysis in private cars. Depending on the type of insurance you carry, whether or not you have a qualifying disability, and your individual circumstances, you may be entitled to medical transportation.

The bad news is that both public and private transportation are not always dependable. I have witnessed some patients either arriving late or having to wait (sometimes over an hour or more) to get their ride home. After four hours in the chair, it makes me very sad to watch any patient having to wait ANY EXTRA TIME for their ride.

ATTITUDE

"I find myself to be about as happy as I make up my mind to be."

Finding out that my kidneys were failing was frightening. All sorts of crazy and mixed up ideas and emotions flooded into my poor brain to the point of overload. I became scared, depressed, and at times was in denial: "This can't be happening to me!" But it was happening, and I quickly realized I had only two choices: accept the reality and deal with it or crumble and give in to whining and depression. I thought about the people I most admired and enjoyed being around, and they weren't the people who constantly complained about their aches and pains or how life was unfair. It was my first step in learning a very important lesson, and one that has changed my life. Happiness is a choice, and I can choose to be happy.

My life and my friendships in particular became all the more precious to me. The last thing I wanted was to have my complaining push away the people I loved. The truth was that when I focused on how others were feeling, it helped me to feel better too. Oprah Winfrey reinforced my focus on gratitude, and I was surprised how profound that one shift was for me. I was soon reading more books and quotes on the subject of attitude including *Attitude of Gratitude* by M.J. Ryan. It is still one of my all time favorite books, and I would encourage you to read it.

As much as I've learned from the books I've read, sometimes other patients have been my best teachers. When I first started treatments, there was a handsome young man who came into the dialysis center the same days I did. It was impossible not notice his warm smile and the cheerful hello he offered to people on his way to his chair. Being one who dreaded going every time, I was incredulous.

One day, I happened to run into him at a local store. After stopping to let him know how much he had impressed me, we began to talk. His name was Frank, and he readily admitted that dialysis was not easy, but that wasn't going to repress his bubbly personality. He'd made his choice to be happy early on. We've been friends ever since that day, and despite being knocked down repeatedly by medical setbacks, he has amazed me over and over again with his ability to bounce back. Frank's kidneys are gone, but he refuses to let anything repress his positive attitude. I will always be grateful for his friendship, his extraordinary spirit, and the joy he has brought to my life.

Along with my friend Frank, other dialysis patients have offered words of encouragement along the way. These are some of my favorites, and I'd like to share them with you:

* You have to choose which road you want to take.

* No one else can do it for you.

* Do not let dialysis be the only thing. Live your life.

* Your life doesn't stop here… it starts.

* It certainly will get easier.

* Do what the doctor tells you <u>when</u> your doctor tells you.

* Don't be afraid to ask questions.

* Every day above the ground is a good day.

* Really… you'll be OK… <u>you can live with this</u>.

* It beats the alternative.

A positive attitude can be cultivated in different ways, but when you find it, nurture it. A strategy I especially like is to make at least three people smile every day, starting with myself. I had always been little a shy, but I decided not to let that get in my way, and now it's just become a natural part of who I am. The truth is, you can't make someone else smile without smiling yourself, and when that happens, it's just hard not to feel better. Besides that, it's fun! I am an equal opportunity smiler, and before I know it, I'm chatting with the grocery clerks, the janitors, and people passing by... whoever happens to cross my path. If I were going to spread something contagious, I'd just as soon make it a smile!

So much more than we realize, happiness is indeed a choice. I choose to be happy when I walk into the dialysis center... not because of the procedure, but because of opportunities it gives me. I get to be with my dialysis buddies, share that smile, or just say hello. The members of the dialysis staff have become my dear friends, and I always enjoy seeing them. I know each one by name and try my best to bring sunshine to their day. They certainly bring that to mine. They work long, hard hours, and their decision to choose the career that they have is a gift of life to every dialysis patient they care for. How could I not be happy to have a chance to be with people like that and to have friends like that? They will never know how much I admire and deeply appreciate each one of them. I don't have enough words of love for these people, and I will be forever grateful that they have become such a special part of my life.

Regular dialysis treatments will always have their ups and downs, and that is just part of the process. None of us can change that, but keeping a positive attitude can help you just as it has me. What a gift it is to know that choice is always yours.

PLANNED DIVERSIONS

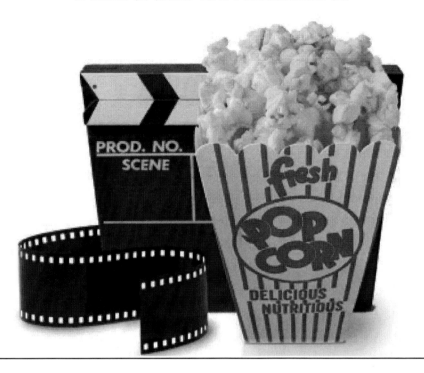

Early in my treatment, I started thinking of going to dialysis just like getting to go to an old fashioned matinee. Of course, you can read, sleep, or watch TV, but I found that having my own DVD player and watching movies was a super way to pass the time. If you don't have your own device, your unit will probably provide a free laptop for your use. You can surf the Internet, play games, or use it to watch all those DVD movies you have been missing. I highly recommend signing up and using a service like *Netflix*® as it can provide you with a constant stream of viewing options. There can be a lot of distractions with machines beeping away and sometimes I have a little difficulty concentrating or I get sleepy. Having a good DVD can diminish the boredom. I always bring along a big bag of unbuttered, unsalted popcorn and enjoy the show.

ADVICE FROM OTHER PATIENTS

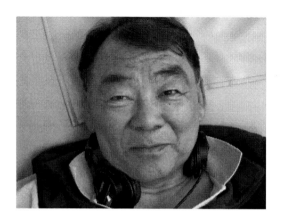

Sungsoo Kim

How long have you been doing dialysis?
Almost eight years.

Why did you choose hemodialysis?
It's more convenient for me to come to the facility where there are professionals.

What was or is the most difficult part for you?
Not being able to take trips or vacations without planning way ahead of time.

What tips, tricks, or advice would you like to share with someone who is about to start dialysis?
Dialysis gives you life. Keeping a good attitude is the most important thing. Sleeping is the easiest way to pass the time. The four hours goes a lot faster that way. In the beginning, I drank too much and was hospitalized. I learned that by drinking less, I have limited the pain that comes with the process of taking off excess fluids.

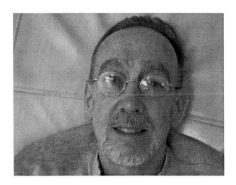

David LePard

How long have you been doing dialysis?
Four years.

Why did you choose hemodialysis?
I just wasn't interested in home dialysis, basically due to lack of knowledge. I'd rather have it done professionally. I feel a little more comfortable than doing it myself.

What was or is the most difficult part for you?
Beginning treatment and the fear of the unknown. People may not admit it, but it's lack of knowledge. Eventually dialysis just becomes a way of life. They don't give you a lot of preparation. You don't know what the experience of dialysis is going to be like for the first two or three months. It's like that with anything.

What tips, tricks, or advice would you like to share with someone who is about to start dialysis?
Visiting a dialysis unit and talking with people before you get started would probably put a lot of people's minds at ease. One thing that was never explained to me was the EMLA cream to numb your arm. It made the first few times quite painful without the cream on my arm. It would have been helpful; nobody told me about that.

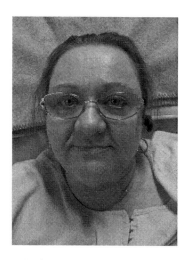

Nancy Dilback

How long have you been doing dialysis?
Almost four years.

Why did you choose hemodialysis?
I wasn't eligible for peritoneal because of previous surgery.

What was or is the most difficult part for you?
Sitting in the chair for five hours. At first, it was difficult having a catheter because I couldn't swim or shower at the gym. Now that I have a fistula, my activities are more open.

What tips, tricks, or advice would you like to share with someone who is about to start dialysis?
Find things to keep you occupied. Make yourself a kit to bring to dialysis including a blanket, things to read, and a couple of snacks. Doing puzzles takes your mind off the time. A telephone is nice too. If you are itching all the time, it's most likely you're not following your dietary instructions. If you just itch when you are having your dialysis, you can ask the technician to start an extra bag of saline through your dialysis filter before you begin, and it will decrease the itching a lot.

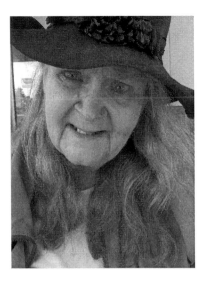

Susi Henderson

How long have you been doing dialysis?
Four years.

Why did you choose hemodialysis?
It seemed a simple way to go about it. It would be harder having dialysis where I live. Coming to the dialysis center is just so much easier, plus I get to go out.

What was or is the most difficult part for you?
The beginning was hard, but now I would say none of it is difficult. Sometimes my transportation is late, and I have to wait a long time to be picked up and taken home.

What tips, tricks, or advice would you like to share with someone who is about to start dialysis?
Find out what your options are and whether you qualify.
Trust in God. Get a good support system going.

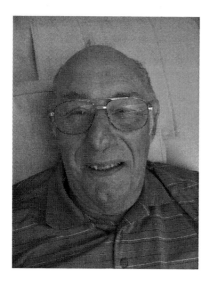

Jim Cook

How long have you been doing dialysis?
Almost three years.

Why did you choose hemodialysis?
Because my doctor told me, "Do it or you'll be dead!"

What was or is the most difficult part for you?
Basically, the four hours sitting on my rear.

What tips, tricks, or advice would you like to share with someone who is about to start dialysis?
I started out with getting the shots of lidocaine in the arm, so they could put the needles in without the pain. Now I use the EMLA cream, which is far better. You put it on an hour before you come, and it is much better than getting the shots all the time.

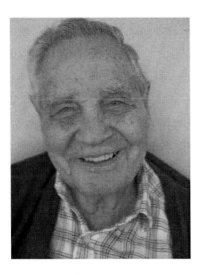

Albert Campbell

How long have you been doing dialysis?
Almost two years.

Why did you choose hemodialysis?
As far as having it done at home, I figured I was too old and forgetful, and so is my wife. We thought about it, but we decided it was better to come in and let the young people take care of me.

What was or is the most difficult part for you?
Sitting here four hours a day, three times a week.

What tips, tricks, or advice would you like to share with someone who is about to start dialysis?
You've got to grin and bear it.

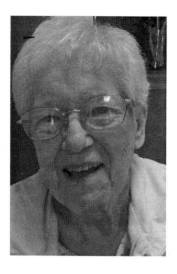

Diane Walsh

How long have you been doing dialysis?
Almost seven years.

Why did you choose hemodialysis?
I think it's a lot easier to let the technicians take care of me rather than doing it myself at home.

What was or is the most difficult part for you?
Coming to dialysis (laughs) three times a week.

What tips, tricks, or advice would you like to share with someone who is about to start dialysis?
Watch the potassium and the sodium. The rest just kind of falls into place. I live in a retirement home and eat most of what they serve, but I do try to stay away from too much potassium and the sodium.

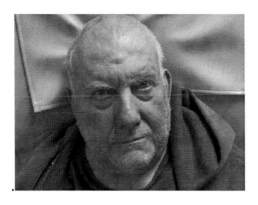

Stanley Terry

How long have you been doing dialysis?
Eight years.

Why did you choose hemodialysis?
My doctor recommended it. I was gaining too much weight, and I had too much water retention to go on peritoneal.

What was or is the most difficult part for you?
Just the time it takes for the procedure. Thank goodness I can sleep through it.

What tips, tricks, or advice would you like to share with someone who is about to start dialysis?
You really do need things to pass away the time. Sleeping, reading, or watching TV works for me.

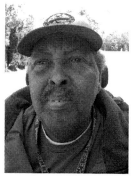

Lacy Wilbon

How long have you been doing dialysis?
Twelve years.

Why did you choose hemodialysis?
Since I'm in a wheelchair, I wanted to be able to get out of the house. It goes better for me if I'm not shut up and confined all the time. I like to be able to get out of the house and go someplace. It makes me feel like I'm going somewhere.

What was or is the most difficult part for you?
Keeping my fluid levels low is hard. I drink too much water and diet soda.

What tips, tricks, or advice would you like to share with someone who is about to start dialysis?
Make taking your medicine a religion. Do what the doctor tells you WHEN your doctor tells you to do it. Get out and be active. Don't sit around and mope. Keep a positive attitude. That's the most important point I can express to you as it just makes everything a whole lot better and easier. Don't be a whiner. I made my mind up that whatever happened, I wasn't going to complain about it. Some people like to have something to complain about. I don't. Take what life gives you and just keep in mind that you are very fortunate to be alive. Every day above the ground is a good day.

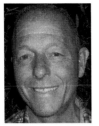

Frank Jones

How long have you been doing dialysis?
Fourteen years.

Why did you choose hemodialysis?
I've chosen to come here to the center because it keeps it separate from my daily life and home.

What was or is the most difficult part for you?
Driving back home from dialysis. Becoming normal again. Sometimes it takes a few hours, sometimes it takes a whole day, and sometimes you don't even notice it happened but when it does, you've got to deal with it.

What tips, tricks, or advice would you like to share?
Having dialysis can be kind of freaky at first but as you go it's fine and you start feeling better, especially if you were feeling bad before you started. For me, itching was an issue. One of the things I found out about scratching your itches is to scratch them backwards. Use the top of your fingernails and instead of digging forward, dig backwards and then your skin doesn't rip and you don't wear out your skin. Concerning fluids, take tiny, little sips. Drink little but swallow a lot. The more you swallow, the more you feel quenched. You can fool your body into thinking you have been drinking a lot. I'll drink a 1/2 cup of water but take as many as 25 sips. Make sure that with every little sip, you get the inside of your mouth and tongue as wet as possible as you swallow.

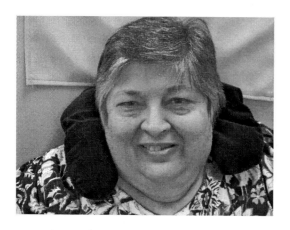

<u>Alberta Duke</u>

How long have you been doing dialysis?
Three years.

Why did you choose hemodialysis?
I looked at peritoneal but didn't have the space at home for it and had no one to watch me. I am a social person, and I like to go to the center.

What was or is the most difficult part for you?
Leg cramps. Sometimes they are quite painful, usually when I take too much fluid off.

What tips, tricks, or advice would you like to share with someone who is about to start dialysis?
My doctor told me it was kind of like taking insulin; nobody wants to do it. But you do it; get a routine, then it is doable. Although this is not for everyone, I find that if I take oxygen, I cramp less. The staff and patients are very nice, and I enjoy talking with them.

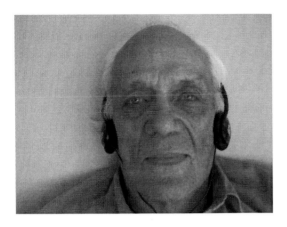

Lyle Anderson

How long have you been doing dialysis?
Six months.

Why did you choose hemodialysis?
The doctor just set me up here.

What was or is the most difficult part for you?
The time involved being sitting still for a long time. Not being able to go out on my boat whenever I want to.

What tips, tricks, or advice would you like to share with someone who is about to start dialysis?
You got to figure out the best way to spend the time.

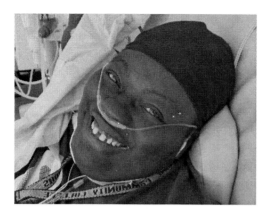

Latina Brooks

How long have you been doing dialysis?
Six months.

Why did you choose hemodialysis?
I work and go to school. At first, it seemed best to come to the center and not have dialysis interfere with my home activities, but now, I've changed my mind, and my next goal is to have dialysis at home.

What was or is the most difficult part for you?
Feeling out of control with my body.

What tips, tricks, or advice would you like to share with someone who is about to start dialysis?
Don't let dialysis be the only thing. Live your life. Your life doesn't stop here... **it starts.**

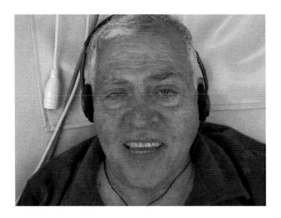

Victor Andrade

How long have you been doing dialysis?
Less than one month.

Why did you choose hemodialysis?
This is what the doctor started me on, so here I am.

What was or is the most difficult part for you?
Putting the needles in. I have what they call eroding veins and it is kind of hard to poke me in the right place. At first there was a lot of bruising, but now it is going a lot better.

What tips, tricks, or advice would you like to share with someone who is about to start dialysis?
The thing that I've learned is that you've got to be on a strict diet and you've got to exercise. I think it is best to start with hemodialysis at the center first, before you start thinking about having peritoneal at home.

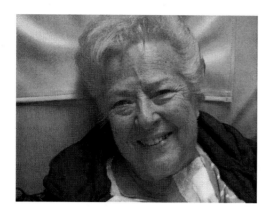

Carole Gilchrist

How long have you been doing dialysis?
Six years.

Why did you choose hemodialysis?
I had to choose something, and I did not like the idea of having a room at home set aside for the treatment. I did not want to involve my husband so intently because it would have. Being able to walk away from the kidney center, go home, and put it behind me is the best for me.

What was or is the most difficult part for you?
When I first started dialysis, I cried all the time and prayed a lot. I was feeling terribly sorry for myself and that was a really big hurdle to get over.

What tips, tricks, or advice would you like to share with someone who is about to start dialysis?
Coming in and volunteering first (before I started) for a few weeks might have helped me. Find something to entertain yourself (besides TV) like visiting with the other patients and technicians. Having a few of your friends come and visit occasionally helps break up the time. It beats the alternative.

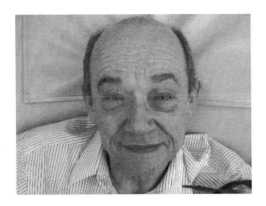

Ward Oakshott

How long have you been doing dialysis?
Almost three years.

Why did you choose hemodialysis?
I tried peritoneal, and hemodialysis worked better. So why give up when something works? I like it a lot better.

What was or is the most difficult part for you?
It's not the dialysis itself, but since I also work, I find that coordinating my work and dialysis is sometimes frustrating. Also, sometimes when I finish dialysis, all I want to do is go home and sleep.

What tips, tricks, or advice would you like to share with someone who is about to start dialysis?
Stay with the diet. I've worked from that, and I've given up some things, and it's all worth it. To me, staying with the diet is the most important thing.

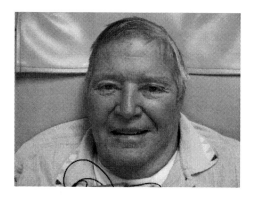

William O'Brien

How long have you been doing dialysis?
Less than a year.

Why did you choose hemodialysis?
My doctor chose it for me. The option for home dialysis didn't present itself. I live in assisted living.

What was or is the most difficult part for you?
It interrupts my schedule and anchors me to a location so that I can't travel anymore. Travel is very restrictive. I've heard that cruise ships have it available, but I don't know much about it. It takes the spontaneity out of travel. I used to have that.

What tips, tricks, or advice would you like to share with someone who is about to start dialysis?
The decision to have dialysis is easy. If you don't have dialysis, you die. Diabetes itself is rather insidious. People don't know what's going on until it's too late. I think people are oblivious to diabetes; they don't want to take action with their diet. Prevention is critical because dialysis is the end result. I should have paid more attention to my diabetes.

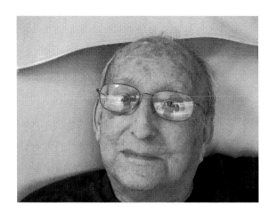

Bob Burrill

How long have you been doing dialysis?
Almost two years.

Why did you choose hemodialysis?
Because of my age, mainly. I also moved from a big house into a small one and have no place to store the supplies needed for peritoneal dialysis.

What was or is the most difficult part for you?
Accepting that I had to be on the machine three days a week. But I did finally accept it, because if you don't accept it, you're just fighting it, and you won't have much of a life doing that. It is difficult to travel because you have to make arrangements far in advance with other kidney centers.

What tips, tricks, or advice would you like to share with someone who is about to start dialysis?
I had my fistula put in two years before starting dialysis. By taking preventative measures with my diet, I was able to delay needing dialysis. The kidney isn't cured with diet, but you can certainly slow down the damage. It HAS to be done and you HAVE to accept that. My relationship with the Lord and knowing He is in charge has made it easier.

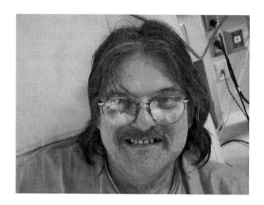

David Roos

How long have you been doing dialysis?
Two years.

Why did you choose hemodialysis?
They wouldn't let me go on home dialysis. I also couldn't do peritoneal dialysis because I had a hernia.

What was or is the most difficult part for you?
Nothing anymore but when I first started it was difficult. It was hard getting here on time. It changes your whole lifestyle. Stop taking in so much fluid; that was the hardest part.

What tips, tricks, or advice would you like to share with someone who is about to start dialysis?
Well, when you get thirsty, instead of drinking water just rinse your mouth out. Just do that four or five times, and you'll quit being so thirsty. It works. I eat popsicles. You'll find out that if you drink too much, it's harder to breathe. I try to stay active. I'm one of the few people that ride a bicycle to dialysis.

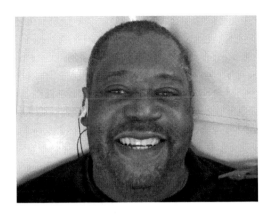

Ronald Thomas

How long have you been doing dialysis?
About a year.

Why did you choose hemodialysis?
I wasn't comfortable with doing it at home.

What was or is the most difficult part for you?
When I first started dialysis I had cramps, but it is getting easier for me. It takes time to get used to it.

What tips, tricks, or advice would you like to share with someone who is about to start dialysis?
I approach dialysis like I did when I used go to work. I have it scheduled for the same time as when I did work and think of it the same way. Like with having a job, you got to be there on time. It gets easier. Listen to your doctor. Really, you'll be OK. You can live with this.

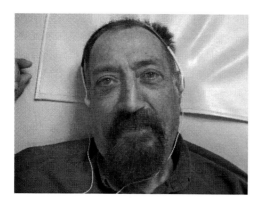

Jesus Marquez

How long have you been doing dialysis?
Two years.

Why did you choose hemodialysis?
I don't like to do it myself, and I don't have the patience to put in the needle and all of that stuff. I'd rather come here and get it done by the professionals.

What was or is the most difficult part for you?
Sitting here for four hours, it gets boring. I read, I watch TV, but sometimes it's still too long for me.

What tips, tricks, or advice would you like to share with someone who is about to start dialysis?
Not to worry about the diet. Eat everything but ONLY a little bit of it. Try to get on with your life. Don't dwell on having to come in all the time. I really appreciate what they do for me here… I'm still alive.

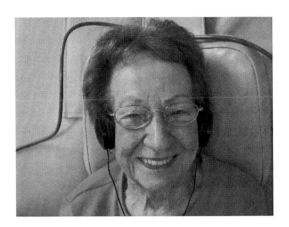

Doreen Spencer

How long have you been doing dialysis?
Four years.

Why did you choose hemodialysis?
I live in a small apartment, and I do not have that much room. I live real close, and it's just so much easier to come here.

What was or is the most difficult part for you?
Preparing food, because there is so much salt in everything you buy. Sometimes I get too much salt.

What tips, tricks, or advice would you like to share with someone who is about to start dialysis?
You just have to take it easy on the days you have dialysis because you're going to be tired afterwards.

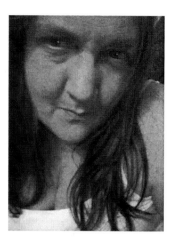

Lisa Elkey

How long have you been doing dialysis?
Eight years.

Why did you choose hemodialysis?
It's much easier to have the professionals do it.

What was or is the most difficult part for you?
Getting up at 4 am. I like getting it over with, so I have the rest of the day to do things.

What tips, tricks, or advice would you like to share with someone who is about to start dialysis?
If I eat before I start the procedure, I feel better. If I don't eat, I sometimes will throw up. I get really bad anxiety, and to keep myself calm, I'll quietly sing. It is hard in the beginning, but it does get easier. The staff is wonderful, and they help a lot.

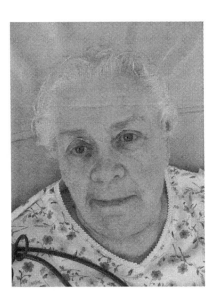

Beverly Young

How long have you been doing dialysis?
One year.

Why did you choose hemodialysis?
I live close to a kidney center. I have many health issues and feel the center is better able to handle the procedure. At home, treatments would put a bigger burden on my family.

What was or is the most difficult part for you?
The hardest part has been getting the fistula to work. After many surgeries, it's finally working beautifully.

What tips, tricks, or advice would you like to share with someone who is about to start dialysis?
Learn everything about you, your health, your diet, and your dialysis. No one else can do it for you. You have to choose which road you want to take. Don't be afraid to ask questions.

POINTS TO REMEMBER

1. Maintain a positive attitude. This is the most important thing that you can do for your own well-being. Be friendly, smile, appreciate the staff, be grateful, and challenge yourself to bring joy into the world. Everyone gets depressed sometimes but it's not fun for anyone to be around constant negativity. YOU can make a difference in someone else's life and inspire others who are facing difficult times too.

2. Create a comfort zone in your chair. A fuzzy blanket and an alternative to TV are musts for me.

3. Try as best you can to stay as close to your "dry weight" between sessions as possible. Reduce your sodium intake. Limiting fluids should be in congruence with how much you are able to urinate. Until the last couple of months, I was able to urinate about 5-6 cups per day, and I drank liquids. Now I only urinate about 2 cups per day and can easily gain 1-2 pounds in the same day, so I have restricted my sodium and liquid intake accordingly. Many patients, especially those who have had their kidneys removed, do not urinate at all and must be much more vigilant about sodium and fluid intake. Watch your diet and think before you drink.

4. Take your medications, especially your phosphorus binders, with every meal. If you are traveling, have your last labs with you and that all-important list of your medications.

5. Always protect your fistula.

6. Become familiar with your lab results and learn from your doctor or dietitian what you might be able to do to improve them. Know what they mean! Learn the terminology and compare each month's results with previous results. Remember, adjust your diet to improve your results or consult with your doctor about additional medications you may need.

7. Listen to your body. It is usually trying to tell you something.

8. Treat too high or too low blood pressure.

9. Avoid getting sick. People with kidney disease have a compromised immune system. You get hit harder than other people by colds, flu, infections, and germs. What starts out as a scratchy throat or cut or scrape can land you in the hospital. The best way to protect yourself is to wash your hands often, avoid people with contagious illnesses, stay current with your immunization shots, and do whatever else you can do to prevent infections. Be sure that your friends and family understand this as well. Protecting you from exposure is by far one of the most important ways they can help and support you.

10. Take advantage of the vast resources of information and guidance available to you. **Some are listed on page 66.**

Resources

Northwest Kidney Centers
http://www.nwkidney.org
206-292-2771

National Kidney Foundation, Inc.
http://www.kidney.org
800-622-9010

Centers for Medicare & Medicaid Services
http://www.medicare.gov
1-800-MEDICARE

DaVita Inc.
http://www.davita.com
303-405-2100

National Kidney and Urologic Diseases Information Clearinghouse
http://kidney.niddk.nih.gov
800-891-5390

Renal Support Network
http://rsnhope.org
818-543-0896

The American Association of Kidney Patients
http://www.aakp.org
800-749-2257

About the author / patient

Kathleen Russell is an artist residing in Seattle, Washington, and is a dialysis patient. She majored in Sociology and Art at the University of LaVerne and spent 20 years in the poster business working with American Arts & Graphics. She has co-written and illustrated several best-selling gift books with her husband Larry Wall. Despite having kidney failure, she continues creating artwork and feeding her three cats.

Watch Kathleen demonstrate and explain her dialysis.

Go to

- SEARCH -
"Dialysis Treatment Procedure"

To order additional copies of this book

Go to...

Also available from

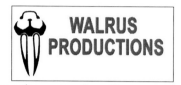

walrusproductions.com

and

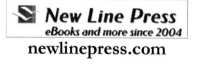

newlinepress.com